Stop Multiple Sclerosis
&
Autoimmune Disease
With high Doses of
Vitamin D

Jennifer Butler

DEDICATION

To all of the fighters out there that knew there must be an answer and who had the courage to never give up!

☐

CONTENTS

INTRODUCTION

I don't believe that it is a mistake that you found this book. Perhaps, someone suggested it. Maybe you accidentally noticed it while browsing titles online or in a bookstore...or my personal favorite, somebody who cares about you shared their copy with you. I don't believe that anything happens by chance. No matter how it crossed your path, the odds are there is a person in your life this book was meant for. Maybe that person is a friend or loved one who you want so badly to help...or maybe that person is you.

When I had proof that vitamin D had halted my disease, I vowed to shout it from the rooftops. Please know, there is so much help between the covers of this book. You can rest assured that I am speaking as a patient who has traveled the same road and is running back as fast as she can to you to say I found a way out! Please follow me, and I will show you how to get there.

I would like to make one request of every person who picks up this book. After you read it please pass it on! This book is not meant to sit on a shelf in pristine condition. This book has a job to do. My wish is that it becomes used, tattered, dog-eared, highlighted and marked up and smudged over and over because it has stayed in motion. It is meant to be shared far and wide with as many as will listen. There will be those that won't. Patience and gentleness can be much more persuasive than constant pressure. Believe me, I get it. When I saw that first MRI free of lesions after 10 years, I wanted to jump out of my chair and drag every patient I could find to the nearest protocol doctor to get them started because I KNEW this worked! I had people say things to me like, "We don't want what you're selling!" It hurt because I wasn't selling anything. In fact, I was running myself ragged trying to get this message out, but how could they know? In a world with a snake-oil salesman around every corner, it is very understandable.

But not everyone can know your heart, and it is normal for people to be skeptical. I was just sharing information and I sincerely wanted to help. After talking to multiple people, I began to realize, however, some of these people have suffered with autoimmune diseases for years. They have tried many of the new promising treatments only to be let down by conventional medicine. Some traveled to other countries and had spent thousands—and in several cases—over a hundred thousand dollars for ineffective therapies. They are very understandably disheartened, angry and afraid to try again. Who could blame them? I'm very blessed with a primary doctor who happens to be a good friend. I was talking to him the other day after learning that a man with MS had been diagnosed with PML. The man commented that he had about 6 to 9 months to live and he was going to fight it every step of the way! His diagnosis made me sad and angry because it does not have to be this way! The pharmaceutical companies look at cases like this as collateral damage, but I look at man, as a man, not an acceptable statistic. He has a family, and they don't consider him collateral damage. They consider him irreplaceable. I told my doctor friend, I get so frustrated because this therapy is so safe and effective, but it is hard to convince people for just that reason. People are dying of PML and no one has died from this treatment! He said, "It is because there is so much snake oil out there, that people are skeptical." He is right. I was one of those people! So please be patient with those that are not ready to hear. I know you love them, and I know how hard it is to watch someone you care about pass up something that can truly help them. What's the old adage? You can lead a horse to water, but you can't make him drink? I heard a wise woman once say, "But you can salt his oats!" I hope to be able to share some salt with you and impart practical information that you can use to help you persuade that person who is afraid and unsure. On the other hand, there are many who will be interested. They will try the therapy, get well, and soon others will see their results. Many times this is the key to getting reticent people to take another look and hopefully one day find out for themselves the freedom from the autoimmune nightmare that this therapy offers.

"The Multiple Sclerosis Foundation estimates that in the United States alone, there are 400,000 cases of multiple sclerosis and about 2.5 million cases worldwide. (Multiple Sclerosis by the Numbers: Facts, Statistics, and You)" "Autoimmune diseases are among the leading causes of death among young and middle-aged women in the United States." (Autoimmune diseases: A leading cause of death among young and middle-aged women in the United States) From what I have learned about the amazing power of vitamin D, I am 100% positive that in the years to come, autoimmune diseases will be discussed as diseases of the past, in the same way that today we discuss ailments such as smallpox, rickets, scurvy, and the plague; a group of diseases that occurred in epidemic proportions until we realized they were triggered by easily-correctable measures. With your help, we can ensure that these diseases are once and for all relegated to the dustbin of history.

In 2007, I was diagnosed with multiple sclerosis. To look at me you would have never known anything was wrong with me at all, but if you could have stepped inside my mind, it would have been difficult to see anything else. There is a joke among MS patients that everyone says, "…but you look so well." For many of us, it is an invisible disease. Many of the symptoms we only feel. The discomfort is very real, but not apparent to the outside world.

It is only the cases of extreme disability that people associate with MS, but the fact is you likely interact with people every day that have MS and you would never know it unless they told you. You cannot see the many ailments that can affect a person with multiple sclerosis such as double vision, spasticity, bowel or bladder issues, sexual dysfunction, vertigo, muscle cramps, cognitive issues, leg weakness, etc. Not everyone has all of these issues, but most people with MS have at least one that is not apparent physically. For me it was mild leg cramps, eye pain, blurry vision, intolerance to heat and a slight numbness along the edge of my left hand. These only occurred every once in a while and none of them were permanent, but all were things that no one could see, but I could feel. There are a myriad of reasons that people choose not to disclose their illness. Some are concerned that it could jeopardize their career. Some are concerned about what it may mean for them socially or in trying to find love. For this reason, the reality is, you walk past people with MS every day and most of the time you will have no idea who they are.

I was one of those people with invisible MS, but if you could take a peek inside my head, you would quickly find that it was a permanent fixture, an ever-present fear of what lie ahead. When I allowed myself to face the reality of what multiple sclerosis meant, it was like a monstrous, impenetrable steel door that slammed shut on my life, my hopes and dreams and for a while, my future. It felt like prison. I have always been a very resourceful person. If a major obstacle presented itself, my choice would always be to fight rather than let my circumstances direct my path, but there was no creative way around this. No amount of hard work would eventually dig me out of it. The disease always wins. You can't beat it. The most you can do is keep it at bay…or so I thought.

I'm here to tell you that I was wrong. So incredibly wrong! There has been a paradigm shift, and it's amazing. I'm asked often why I do what I do. My question is, "How can you not tell people about this?" This is huge! I want everyone to know, not only can you stop your illness in its tracks, but you can help prevent this from ever happening again to those coming up behind you. You will understand by the end of this book that you can be are part of something life changing!

There is hope. Lots and lots of hope. I'm here to show you that you can fling that door wide open and where there was darkness there is nothing but light. Please read on. I promise you won't be disappointed. Right here is where I give you a big hug and tell you friend to friend, it really is going to be okay.

In November of 2015, I learned of a Brazilian Professor of neurology who had developed a treatment for autoimmune diseases and—who at the time had, together with his colleagues—treated approximately 4,000 patients.

Thanks to social media, the news has spread across the world, and as patients share, the news is exploding. I want this book to arm you with information that you can use to explain what vitamin D is and how it halts autoimmune diseases. I will share with you what the protocol is and how to get started. I will explain the fear of vitamin D toxicity (hypercalcemia) that most doctors fear unnecessarily. I will share my personal testimony and the testimonies of others with you. I will share my radiology reports and before and after MRIs, and then offer you some good tips on how to convince those people in your life who are having a hard time believing that a vitamin can do what conventional medicine cannot.

Are you ready? Okay! Let's get started!

ACKNOWLEDGMENTS

Thanks first and foremost to God, for without Him none of this would have been possible.

To my daughter, who did not always understand why mommy could not play as much as she would have liked during the months when I was writing this book.

To my awesome son and writer, Jordan Butler, who listened to me go on and on about vitamin D all the time and kept me sane and laughing during the process of writing this book. You taught me quite a bit about writing; many of those suggestions were put to use in this book.

To my best friend Amy, who sat and listened to me complain about everything for the last 4 years with constant support and no judgement. Thank you for traveling with me to Florida amidst delayed flights, and every possible travel disaster that could have arisen. Because you were with me, we laughed until we cried in circumstances where had you not been there, I'm sure I would have just cried.

To Raven who calmed my fears about MS when I was first diagnosed and has become one of my closest friends through this journey. You are an amazing person and you deserve only the best!

To Chrissy who just jumped in with both feet and helped me steer the ship when the waves of my life were crashing all around me so that the group could continue even when I was unable to be there for a time. You were a pillar of support, a sounding board; always giving gentle and honest feedback and much laughter (I have two words for you: Gorilla Glue!)! You have been such a ray of light to all of us. It was no accident that you showed up.

To the international group leaders who helped us get started and were so gracious to help us with translation so we could understand and help our English-speaking members learn of this amazing treatment!

To my medical team who supported my decisions. The path could have been so much more difficult without your willingness to support me in making the decisions I felt I needed to make and giving me the space to do so.

To our amazing group of men and women who stand shoulder to shoulder against this disease every day. We all feel that we have a common thread and our only goal is to help one another and share this miracle with as many as we can. On a daily basis you humble me with your kindness and make me smile with your love and humor. We all have muddled through this together willing to experiment on ourselves to make way for those that will come after us. Bless you all for your courage. I am so thankful that you trusted us to walk with you on this leg of your journey and if we ever part, go knowing you all will hold one of the most special places in my heart forever.

Lastly, but certainly not least, to Dr. Cicero Galli Coimbra, your pure desire to help each individual patient at the level of their need instead of bowing to convention is commendable. I'm sure your struggles have been many, and no one can ever know what you have suffered as a result. However, I can understand and share the joy that comes each time another patient is reaches that moment when they realize that this is working! Your work is changing lives all over the world and no amount of gratitude will ever be enough to thank you for what you have done.

CHAPTER ONE

HOW CAN A VITAMIN HALT AUTOIMMUNE DISORDERS?

The greatest obstacle to discovery is not ignorance - it is the illusion of knowledge.

-Daniel J. Boorstin

When you tell people that you've been able to halt your multiple sclerosis or other autoimmune disorder with vitamin D, their first question is usually, "How can a vitamin halt MS?" This is an understandable reaction to what, on its face, seems like a claim that's too good to be true. It's a fair question. Once you understand the concepts behind it, however, it unveils a beautiful mosaic created from the pieces of a historically difficult puzzle. One objective of this book is to try sort out those pieces that lay the groundwork for the masterpiece that we know it to be in an easy-to-understand format that gives you the confidence to explain it to friends, loved ones and physicians.

So, how can a vitamin halt autoimmune disorders?

To answer this question well, we need to first understand that vitamin D is actually not a "vitamin" at all. According to Colorado State University VIVO Pathophysiology, "Bioactive vitamin D or calcitriol is a steroid hormone (secosteroid) that has long been known for its important role in

1

regulating the body's levels of calcium and phosphorus, and in mineralization of bone. More recently, it has become clear that receptors for vitamin D are present in a wide variety of cells, and that this hormone has biologic effects which extend far beyond the control of mineral metabolism.

The term vitamin D is, unfortunately, an imprecise term referring to one or more members of a group of steroid molecules. Vitamin D3, also known as cholecalciferol, is generated in the skin of animals when light energy is absorbed by a precursor molecule 7-dehydrocholesterol. Vitamin D is thus not a true vitamin, because individuals with adequate exposure to sunlight do not require dietary supplementation.

There are also dietary sources of vitamin D, including egg yolk, fish oil and a number of plants. The plant form of vitamin D is called vitamin D2 or ergosterol. However, natural diets typically do not contain adequate quantities of vitamin D, and exposure to sunlight or consumption of foodstuffs purposefully supplemented with vitamin D are necessary to prevent deficiencies.

Vitamin D, as either D3 or D2, does not have significant biological activity. Rather, it must be metabolized within the body to the hormonally-active form known as 1, 25-dihydroxycholecalciferol. This transformation occurs in two steps, the first in the liver and the final step in the kidney." At this point the 1, 25(OH) 2D travels through the body attaching itself to vitamin D receptors through the body giving direction for gene expression.

VITAMIN D RECEPTORS (VDR)

With the finding of the vitamin D receptor (VDR) in nearly every tissue and the more recent discovery of thousands of VDR binding sites throughout the genome controlling hundreds of genes, the interest in vitamin D and its impact on multiple biologic processes has accelerated tremendously as evidenced by the thousands of publications each year for the past several years.

Dr. Coimbra describes it this way, "Today we are absolutely convinced, along with the scientific community that deals with research of vitamin D—which studies the effects of vitamin D in the immune system—that vitamin D is the major regulator of the immune system and modifies the operation of approximately 4,500 genes in every cell of the immune system. It is a substance without equal. The lack of this substance is a disaster for the immune system!

Considering VDR binding sites have been located in including the intestine, liver, pancreatic beta cells, epithelial cells, bronchial epithelial cells, skin epithelial cells, osteoblasts and chondrocytes (bone), muscle, immune system, endocrine glands, brain tissue and reproductive tissue, it's easy to see how vitamin D has such a dramatic effect on our entire body and many of its functions. (Biophysics)

HOW CAN VITAMIN D STOP ALL AUTOIMMUNE DISEASES?

Vitamin D suppresses the Th17 response of the immune system that aggravates autoimmune diseases. Autoimmune diseases are all created by this abnormal response. The only known substance that can selectively impede this response is vitamin D. It also has the amazing ability to accomplish this without obstructing other important immune system functions. Furthermore, vitamin D enhances the immune system's ability to fight viruses and bacteria as well as other microorganisms.

"The Th17 reaction is caused by overproduction of an "immune messenger" (cytokine) called "interleukin 17". Production of interleukin 17 is a natural phenomenon and is beneficial in adequate, regulated amounts. However, overproduction of interleukin 17 is not a natural phenomenon. And vitamin D regulates this interleukin 17 production.

So autoimmune disease is the result of a dysregulated immune system that produces an aberrant immunological Th17 reaction. And vitamin D is the substance needed to regulate the immune system."

CHAPTER TWO

HOW WAS THIS TREATMENT DISCOVERED?

"Neurology was this discipline of great diagnosticians,

and yet they had no real answers to any of the most devastating neurological diseases."

-Cicero Galli Coimbra

This treatment was developed by Dr. Cicero Galli Coimbra, MD, PhD. After completing his clinical training in the United States, he returned to São Paolo, Brazil with the intention of researching mouse models of neurological illnesses. Dr. Coimbra states, "In research, we are obligated to be at the forefront. One cannot simply read neurological textbooks and studies from 5 or 10 years ago; one must know what has been published last week that is relevant to the research that one is doing.

Possessing an enormous quantity of research that has not been published in textbooks, we asked ourselves why this information had not been applied in clinical practice; and sometimes this is really basic information. Slowly we became personally convinced that patients would benefit from many things that are not discussed at medical conventions and read in textbooks simply because they can reduce the consumption of pharmaceuticals above all when these medications are costly." (Cicero Galli Coimbra) Dr. Coimbra and his colleagues became convinced that vitamin D triggered the generation of many neuroregenerative components in the brains of everyone from fetuses to adults.

He and his colleagues began treating patients with neurodegenerative diseases with physiologically realistic doses of vitamin D; 10,000 IU, the same as you would get from 10 to 20 minutes in the sun with arms and legs exposed. Dr. Coimbra and his colleagues noticed that one of these patients with Parkinson's disease had a vitiligo lesion on his face and upon return 3 months later the lesion had markedly diminished. This prompted them to research the medical literature for more information. Their research uncovered an enormous amounts of information already out there, and this surprised them. They begin to implement the treatment in patients with multiple sclerosis and were amazed at the great improvement seen in these patients.

Dr. Coimbra states that "Today we are absolutely convinced—along with the scientific community that researches vitamin D—vitamin D is the major regulator of the immune system."

☐

CHAPTER THREE

HOW ARE AUTOIMMUNE DISEASES ACTIVATED?

"The mind most effectually works upon the body, producing by his passions and perturbations miraculous alterations... cruel diseases and sometimes death itself".

Robert Burton, the Anatomy of Melancholy

There are many hypotheses as to what triggers the autoimmune response. Some of the theories involve an acquired infection at an early age such as EBV (Epstein - Barr virus), environmental triggers, a tick bite, processed foods, etc. The list of possible causes is long and many theories are out there. Most agree that the autoimmune response has many components. According to Dr. Coimbra there are three that major causative elements that are notably present in nearly every case.

RESISTANCE

Many times when I speak to people about MS and autoimmune diseases. I explain that people with autoimmune diseases are deficient in vitamin D. invariably, someone will say, "Well, I live in Florida, Arizona, etc., so that cannot be." So I think it is important to say that vitamin D deficiency is not just caused by insufficient sunlight, but in many cases a partial resistance to vitamin D, occurring in different degrees from person to person. According to Dr. Coimbra, "There is an inherited, partial resistance to the biological effects of vitamin D, and limited quantities this powerful modulator predispose people with this genetic resistance to the occurrence of autoimmune diseases."

INSUFFICIENT SUN EXPOSURE

Someone commented to me one time that they felt that it was ironic that at the time of their diagnosis they were encouraged to stay out of the sun and avoid exercise. And as it turns out, those are two of the most important things we may be able to do to prevent this disease. The vitamin D-producing warmth of the sun and the stress-relieving benefits of exercise, might very well prevent the genetic cascade of events that trigger MS. The biggest source of vitamin D is from the sun.

When an adult wearing a bathing suit or a tank top and shorts (arms and legs exposed), lying horizontally, is exposed to one minimal erythemal dose (causing a slight pinkness to the skin 24 hours after exposure of UV radiation), the amount of vitamin D produced is between 10,000 IU and 25,000 IU.

It is well known that the further you go away from the equator, the higher the prevalence of MS. this is believed to be due to the amount of sunlight that these areas receive as far as intensity and due to seasonal fluctuations. There is very little disagreement over this fact today. The less sunshine you get, the less vitamin D your body manufactures.

We have all been told for years to stay out of the sun and to wear sunscreen whenever we are outdoors. Although, skin cancer is a real concern, 10 to 20 minutes in the sun before applying sunscreen is needed to get the vitamin D your body requires as your body only absorbs the vitamin D it needs during this time period.

There has also been quite a bit of discussion lately regarding vitamin D as a protective agent against skin cancer. Some hypothesize that the first 20 minutes you spend in the sun without sunscreen could have a protective effect against skin cancer as well as other cancers.

We absorb vitamin D when the UVB rays of the sun reach our most outer layer (dermis) of the skin, and trigger a chemical decomposition or separation of molecules by the action of light. This process is called photolysis. This happens to a chemical in the skin that is called 7-dehydrocholesterol, thus producing the precursor vitamin D. This vitamin D attaches to a binding protein which then transports the D to the liver. Once in the liver, through a process called hydroxylation, it becomes known by several names, including the most well-known: calcitriol, activated vitamin D or 25(OH)D.

The vitamin D is not active here but all of your tissues, at this point, are able to utilize it and turn it in to 1,25(OH)2D or activated vitamin D because now it is prepared to be utilized by our body. When 25(OH)D is transformed to 1,25(OH)2D in the kidneys it circulates in your blood and maintains the proper calcium balance in our blood.

STRESS

Worry and stress affects the circulation, the heart, the glands, the whole nervous system, and profoundly affects heart action.
– Charles W. Mayo, M.D.

"Stressful life events precede 85% of RRMS relapses! It is acknowledged as, by far, the most important triggering factor of relapses." The World Health Organization suggests that by the year 2030 depression and stress-related problems will be the most debilitating and widespread health disorders on the planet, closely followed (rather tellingly) by autoimmune disease and allergy."

A 2014 review article in the Journal of Immunology states, "…four fundamental emotional responses: anger, anxiety, laughter and relaxation are able modulate cytokine production and cellular responses to a variety of immune stimuli. These modulations are shown to be either detrimental or beneficial to a patient's health dependent on the context and duration of the emotion.

"I am strongly convinced that the increase in autoimmune disease prevalence mainly depends upon three factors" states, Dr. Coimbra. "Some carry this genetic predisposition to autoimmune disorders but do not develop - or have not yet developed – autoimmunity. We believe that something else is necessary in addition to that genetic predisposition to trigger those diseases.

The most consistent, I would even say probably ubiquitous triggering factor in relapsing remitting MS, since we have found almost no exceptions among thousands of patients with autoimmune diseases, is a stressful life event, or a prolonged stressful period – for instance, related to professional or familial environment. It seems to work very similar in most autoimmune disorders.

CHAPTER FOUR

WHY IS THIS NEWS NOT EVERYWHERE?

"By saying it is toxic, you're acknowledging that it is potent and effective."

– Dr. Reinhold Vieth

This was my first question!

...and I'm not the only one who wanted to know this. The question we hear from new members is: "If this is such a great therapy, why are we just hearing about this now?" Word of mouth is powerful, and there definitely is a groundswell of patients thanks to the introduction of numerous Facebook pages dedicated to getting the word out, but we still have much work to do before it becomes mainstream.

The main purposes of this book is to share this life-changing treatment with as many people as we can. One of the greatest obstacles to reaching the population is simply the result of years of conditioning of the medical community to only see one way of doing things where new medical breakthroughs are concerned.

Without a clinical trial, few are willing to even consider such a therapy—even when the proof is right in front of them in the form of a previously-disabled patient with an amazing lack of disability compared to prior exams or an incredibly-telling inactive MRI over subsequent studies, after years of active lesions and progression.

Yes, MS can quiet down sometimes, but when patients continue to improve and show no more signs of decline, it's very hard to refute. Clinical trials are nearly impossible due to the ethics of it in cases such as these. We are talking about a seriously debilitating illness. Giving a patient a placebo in this case would be unethical.

If a person has a diagnosed disorder that could be harmful or potentially fatal, the doctor is obligated to try and correct that. For instance, in a situation where a patient has some sort of deficiency a conscientious physician understands that he has a responsibility to correct or modify treatment to the benefit of the patient. To ask a doctor to do otherwise, would be to expect the doctor to turn his or her back on the needs of the patient.

For this reason a randomized double-blind study has never been performed. The question is one of the ethical treatment of the patient. How do you justify giving one group a proven therapy that would help them while leaving the second group to languish on a placebo? This would leave the patients open to further disability when the doctor knows that he could help them. This is incongruent with the promise the doctor made when he began to practice medicine to first do no harm.

The medical community today believes that published results cannot be given consideration if they have not first resulted from a randomized double-blind study, and therein lies the problem. It has been my experience since I have been working with the members of my Facebook group, Coimbra Vitamin D Protocol for MS & Autoimmune Disorders that a member will discuss this therapy with their physician or neurologist in order to get the needed baseline labs drawn that are required to begin the protocol. However, due to the fear of vitamin D toxicity (hypercalcemia) or other contributing factors or influences, the physician, out of a lack of knowledge, fear of liability and several other factors is unwilling to help implement the treatment.

Because of this, the patient then, out of frustration and an inability to find help, decides to begin the protocol on his own through a protocol doctor. In the majority of instances—Dr. Coimbra cites about 95% of the time—the treatment is highly successful (success is considered 100% disease suppression), and so when the patient returns to his physician with marked improvements physically and evidenced by inactive lesions on MRI, this is the point at which doctors begin to take notice. Most protocol doctors are born out of these experiences.

CHAPTER FIVE

AREN'T THESE DOSES TOXIC?

Without the supervision of a protocol doctor, yes, vitamin D can produce toxicity as a result of attempting to implement the protocol independent of medical supervision using high doses, using supplements from an unreliable source, hyperthyroidism and excessive consumption of vitamin C. For this reason, the Coimbra Protocol requires monitoring by a trained protocol provider. Additionally, a person with an autoimmune disease, having a partial resistance to vitamin D to varying degrees, requires more vitamin D to compensate for that resistance.

The major concern with vitamin D toxicity is hypercalcemia or excess calcium, which can result in calcification of the arteries, heart, as well as kidney stones or in severe cases renal failure. This problem is controlled by the restriction of dairy products and some high-calcium foods. We all need some calcium in our diets, but the excess calcium is unnecessary.

We drink a minimum of 2.5 liters of liquid per day to dilute and flush any excess calcium—which is found in nearly every food—through our kidneys in the urine.

Patients on the protocol are required to get routine lab testing at regular intervals to ensure they remain within safe ranges. It is a very simple diet and the restrictions are few. Most dairy products have very palatable alternatives and so once you get the hang of the diet you really don't feel as though you are sacrificing anything. Most importantly, you are gaining your health!

CALCIUM RESTRICTION AND BONE HEALTH

Our bodies need calcium for many different functions. We think of calcium as the mineral that forms bone and teeth, but it is also responsible for muscle contraction, normal functioning of many enzymes, blood clotting and normal heart rhythm.

Calcium is extremely important for many of our body systems. We get calcium from two sources: our food and our bones. If we do not get enough calcium from our food, our body will obtain it from our bones and this is what concerns many physicians.

However, what many people are unaware of is that you can build bone density through weight bearing activities such as weight training, walking, hiking, jogging, climbing stairs, tennis, running, jumping walking lunges, and dancing, which do an excellent job of not only maintaining, but building bone density. Any movement that requires the pushing and pulling of the bones and muscles against gravity make good weight bearing activities.

When you bear weight, it signals your body to form more bone. There is an interesting phenomena called spaceflight osteoporosis where astronauts, not having gravity to cause resistance in the bones and muscles, typically lose more bone mass during one month in space than postmenopausal women on Earth lose in one year. Weight bearing exercise is very important!

For those who are unable to engage in these activities, you'll be happy to know that many people have found great success with vibration boards according to several studies.

In my own experience, I have found weight bearing exercise to cause an increase in my bone density when I exercised, and noted a decrease when I did not. During my first 6 months on the treatment, when the weather was warm I walked on average about 30 to 45 minutes daily. My DEXA scan showed an increase in my bone density. However, during the next 6-month period, when the weather was colder and I did not get out as often, my DEXA showed a decrease in bone density. For this reason, part of the protocol is to walk at least 30 minutes 5 days a week.

For those who are unable to do this initially, a vibration board may be a very good investment. They are FDA approved and so should be covered by Medicaid for patients whom financial constraints are a concern. Some patients are prescribed medications to protect against osteoporosis if they are unable to exercise—or at least until they can exercise. Everyone is different, but many mobility issues can be overcome with creative solutions and proper equipment.

CHAPTER SIX

FINDING OUT

Stress has been a part of my life for as long as I can remember; much of it situational. I managed the circumstances I was unable to change to the best of my ability. In 2005, I moved to Arizona and made a concerted effort to get back into shape. I lost 50 pounds. I was walking several miles a day in the hot Arizona sun and I felt great! One evening before work I came down with a paralyzing exhaustion that I could not shake. It felt as if someone had injected me with an extremely-powerful sedative. I've heard it described before as a feeling of "lie down or fall down." It was not your run-of-the-mill, long-day kind of tired. It was pure exhaustion. It was I-can-barely-lift-my-arms kind of tired.

I did not know what was going on at the time. I chalked it up to being in the sun too long that day, but in retrospect, I realize now it was very likely MS fatigue. I had never felt anything like that before, and I knew I could not make it across the room let alone to work.

Looking back now, I believe I have had symptoms all the way back to my 20s. When I was 21, I went to help my husband's friend set up our Christmas tree. He asked me to help hold the trunk of tree so he could center it. I went to grip the trunk of the tree and could not grip it. It was like my hand just forgot how to carry out the steps to grip something. I told my hand what to do, but my hand could not carry out the instructions. I tried to squeeze my fingers together, but they just would not operate. It only lasted seconds, but that was such a strange experience that I never forgot it.

What I think was my second episode occurred during another period of extreme stress. My eye developed a twitch that lasted for a month. I thought it was stress related but knowing what I know now, I suspect this was an early MS symptom (The Lancet Neurology).

I came back to Virginia from Arizona in the fall of 2006. The stress in my life continued. My old habits along with the weight began to creep back. Several months after coming home, we were faced with several very stressful family issues. One of these issues was the revelation that my mother-in-law was suffering from Alzheimer's disease and had to be moved from her home. Due to some decisions that were made hastily by other family members, we had to move the entire house (a lifetime of things) in a matter of days. My husband was working 2 full-time jobs, 7 days a week. I was raising a child, taking care of a home and working. We were both exhausted physically and mentally, and neither of us had any spare time.

Due to the short notice and our already razor-thin schedules, we were left scrambling to remove the contents of a home—a lifetime of possessions—and find a place to put them in 3 days! Because my husband (then boyfriend) could not get time off of work, we had only had a few hours a day to work on this, and 3 days to accomplish the entire project. It was a monumental task, and the fact that this was on a very hot, humid week in the late spring did not help matters.

On the second day, we worked hard all afternoon in the heat and humidity. I was really out of shape, and compared to my physical endurance level today, I really could not do very much. I was so easily winded. I could feel myself becoming increasingly exhausted but kept pushing myself until I could do no more. I decided I had to take a break before I passed out.

At that point I was standing on the back of a flatbed trailer loading boxes onto it. I'm not sure what possessed me to do it, but I chose to jump off the back of the trailer, about 4 feet from the ground. I hadn't done anything like that in years and being overweight, it really jarred me when I hit the ground. I immediately felt a jolt in my head. When I turned around to look over my right shoulder, I got an odd dizzy sensation. I thought it would go away, but it didn't. Slowly but surely the dizziness got worse. As the day went on, I became increasingly concerned, and told my husband and brother-in-law how to assess for a stroke should I start acting oddly because my suspicion was that what I was feeling were the beginning signs of a stroke, but I dismissed it and continued to help them move. After all, we were under rigid time constraints, and I did not want to hold us up.

The next morning, I woke up with double vision. The only way that I could see correctly was if I would close one eye. If both eyes were open, I saw two equal pictures of everything in front of me, like a side by side computer monitor setup. I thought it was due to eye strain because my work had me in front of a computer screen for 8 to 10 hours a day.

I made an appointment with an eye doctor. He suggested I get a pair of sunglasses and put a patch inside one lens so that no one could tell, and it would obscure the vision in the second eye allowing me to only see one image. I used the patch, but it was difficult to get it to stay in place, and I found it more of a distraction than anything else. Closing one eye worked better for me. So I closed one eye and worked several more days that way.

I did not get checked out because I was afraid they would tell me that I would have to stop working, and I needed to work. I drove with one eye closed and did fine, until one evening when I was backing out of a parking spot and looked over my right shoulder and my vision problems combined with my dizziness resulted in my misjudging my distance, and I almost backed into a woman's car. That scared me, and I began to consider getting checked out.

My husband's friend had requested that I help him sell some tires on EBay. He had never done it before and wanted to learn. We were to go to the UPS hub that evening to send them to the buyer. I drove across town in traffic with one eye closed to meet him there. I could see perfectly with one eye closed, but it got tiring having to squint that eye for so long. My husband's friend asked if I was okay to drive home, and I told him that I was. However, he suggested we call his wife who worked for an eye doctor. She seemed concerned and suggested I go to the emergency room. So instead of going home, I went to the hospital. I figured they would tell me to rest that eye, which would most likely mean not working, but it was obvious it was not going away and I really needed to have this checked out.

I went to the emergency room. They asked me questions as to how this all came about. I still thought I jarred something in my head and that was the reason for all of this. I was certain that's what it was, because that is the exact moment the dizziness began. I had to do a series of neurological tests, a CT scan and ultimately an MRI.

I was in the emergency room all night. It was cold and on that particular night the emergency room was empty—something rare for an

ER.

I was there alone, and as patients were discharged or moved up to the floor one by one. The emergency room became eerily quiet, with only the occasional sound of beeps and buzzes. You could've heard a pin drop in there that night, and because of this I could hear everything the doctors were saying. At one point I heard them say three possible things that may be wrong with me: multiple sclerosis, a brain tumor, and something else that I don't recall.

I remember the words "brain tumor" because they terrified me. They immediately conjured up images of chemo and sickness and thoughts of who would help me take care of my son. He was 8 then, and my husband was always working. I had no family close.

Multiple sclerosis was the last thing on my mind because I had been healthy all my life. I was rarely ill. I never needed pain medication after surgical procedures, I healed very quickly. I rarely caught illnesses when people around me were ill. Seriously! I thought I was Superwoman. I was about to learn differently.

At this point, I still thought they were wasting their time because I was sure this was the result of my jumping off that trailer. I did not have anything that would signal to me multiple sclerosis. However I really didn't know anything about multiple sclerosis. All I knew was it was that disease where people wind up in a wheelchair. I had no trouble walking.

I did not understand why I had been there all night and there was no sign of my being discharged anytime soon. I had gotten there around 5 p.m., and it was now 3 a.m. At some point I fell asleep. I woke up around 5 a.m. in a hospital room. I had been admitted!

I was beginning to become concerned. What was going on? About 5 a.m. I was awakened by a nice, young female doctor who was doing morning rounds. She had a gaggle of students who followed her in. They all huddled over to the side of the room watching our interaction intently with their notes in hand. She introduced herself as the neurologist on duty that morning. She performed the test with the red flashing light that I had become so accustomed to. She asked me several questions.

I remember one student in the back asking, "Is she always going to be like this?" and that scared me because I didn't realize how bad my diagnosis was going to be. I looked down and assessed my body searching for whatever it was that this girl saw. Everything looked normal. Then I realized, this girl knew what was wrong with me. All of them knew, but I was still in the dark. It annoyed me somehow. Shouldn't I be the first to know? I understand now that when they round, they give the students a brief synopsis of what is going on and explain to them the tests they may perform on the patient, but I was pretty scared and hypersensitive after waiting all night in the emergency room, hearing the doctors and nurses discussing my possible diagnoses. We like to feel in control of our lives, but I felt anything but in control at that moment. I felt completely helpless.

When the doctor returned around noon, I had still had no idea what was going on. However when she slowly walked over and pulled up a chair, I instantly knew she was not going to be giving me good news. I didn't want to hear what she had to say. I was waiting for the brain tumor talk. Boy! Did she catch me off guard! She sat down and very matter-of-factly said, "We think you have multiple sclerosis." I thought, "That's crazy, I just jumped off a truck!" I could not understand how they could come to that conclusion. I was stunned. I wanted to ask her questions because I really thought she was wrong but I just couldn't summon the strength to utter the words. She was compassionate, but to the point, and I appreciated her directness.
☐

A NEW NORMAL

That is one of the moments of my life that will be etched in my brain forever. I say I was strong, but I think I was just numb. I was definitely in shock. In retrospect, I think shock and numbness are amazing protective tactics our minds and bodies use to rescue us in situations like this. They are like two big arms that sweep you up right before the fall. They protect you until your mind can handle it. I was thankful for those amazing safety mechanisms God provides us with to be able to handle blows such as the one I had just received.

I went through all of the emotions that you see people go through. This must be a mistake? After all, I knew what I felt, and I felt a jolt to my head the second I jumped off that trailer, and the minute I turned around the dizziness started. In the back of my head I really didn't believe it. I don't even think it was denial because of how coincidental it was. So I asked, "How sure are you?" She said, "65% to 75% sure." Of course, me being the eternal optimist, thought, "Okay, so there is a 25% to 35% chance they're wrong." I went with that. It was all I had that I could hang on to, so I took it!

I really knew nothing about MS. In my mind, I pictured myself at some point in the near future in a wheelchair with twisted limbs, unable to care for myself. That thought absolutely terrified me. It's this thought that terrifies anyone with MS.

When I sat there in the hospital bed and the doctor had given me the news, and asked if I had any questions. I could feel a lump forming in my throat. I was fighting back tears and thought back to an old friend that battled cancer with humor and grace and a promise I had made to myself that if I was ever diagnosed with something as significant as cancer, I would want to handle it the way she did. With dignity. I did not want anyone feeling sorry for me. I wanted to be an inspiration to others. I could decide right then and there whether I was going to allow it to consume me or whether I was going to go down fighting. I chose the latter.

When the doctor asked if I had any questions, I said, "Yes. So I straightened myself up in bed, very stoic, and thought for a minute. Finally, I calmly said, "Okay, I have three questions…" My first question was "Will I end up in a wheelchair?" Her answer, "Most likely, no, but we can't predict the course." The second questions was, "How long will my lifespan be?" Her answer was, "About the same as anyone else." I could die a bit earlier of complications from MS, e.g. pneumonia, etc., but no one could predict that. Most likely I would live a full life. The third question was so difficult I saved it until the end. "Could I have passed this on to my son?" Thankfully her answer was, "No, not likely." There was a slim chance in our genetic code he would have the possibility of developing it, but probably no more than anyone else. It is a mix of the potential gene combination for autoimmunity combined with a lot of outside environmental factors. Once I learned that, I felt like I could handle everything else.

She handed me a big purple and white binder and told me to go home and look through it. The purple and white kit was very large and clunky. It was filled with information about the drug that she felt was best suited for what I had. I was diagnosed with relapsing-remitting multiple sclerosis (RRMS). It is the type of MS that most people begin with. You have relapses and then the disease remits. You can have complete recovery or not. After some point, most people transition to a more progressive form of the disease.

The kit contained things like a notebook, a video, a chart where you could write down when you took your shot and where you injected, e.g. "right arm", "left leg", etc. It was advised that you rotate the injection site between your arms and legs each time. The drug was called Avonex (interferon beta-1a). It was a large 1.25-gauge needle. It was the only one of the 4 CRAB (Copaxone, Rebif, Avonex and Betaseron) drugs that had to be administered intramuscularly so the needle had to be long enough to go through my skin and deep enough to get into the muscle. The other three were given subcutaneously (just beneath the skin).

One of the more positive aspects of Avonex was that it was less likely than the others to develop neutralizing antibodies or antibodies that render the medication ineffective. It only worked in about a third of the patients, and the relapse reduction rate was just over 30%. I did not feel very confident about this drug's efficacy and wondered just exactly what benefit I was actually getting. I kept hearing, we didn't have any drugs, and now we have four. Yes, but how effective were they really?

Later, they came out with other medications that were more effective, but with even more dangerous side effects; one of them a brain virus progressive multifocal leukoencephalopathy (PML), which took the lives of 3 people before being taken off the market. There was little to entice one to choose these. It was just the only choice, so what else could you do? It appeared the choices were to get worse or to take one of these extremely-expensive, minimally-effective drugs with a high rate of side effects. The drugs, for most, were just the lesser of two evils. I would be injecting into myself weekly for the rest of my life.

I had to give myself an in injection in the arms or the legs once a week to try to keep my disease under control. In some cases it would reduce the rate of relapse and in others it did not. It honestly did not inspire a lot of confidence. The neurologist wanted me to go to the infusion center to get an intravenous Solu-Medrol (IVSM) infusion as soon as possible. This is an extremely high dose of steroids given by IV for an hour over the course of 3 days. Its sole purpose is to shut down the inflammation in the brain that is causing your current flare.

I went to the hospital and was led up to the infusion center, where people receive intravenous infusions; many of them for chemotherapy. The nurse took me in to a tiny room with a bunch of chairs that looked like the type you would see in a dentist's office arranged in sort of a half circle. I think the idea was that people would converse with one another. Most of the people in there were thin and pale with thinning hair, no hair or with headscarves on. Here I was young, full of energy with a head full of long, thick, curly hair. I felt so bad every time I had to go to the infusion center because I knew that some of these people were terminally ill, and I just had MS. It made me realize how lucky I was. I thought, "So what if I did end up in a wheelchair?" I will still see my daughter graduate. I can watch her walk down the aisle, and I can certainly hold my grandkids from a wheelchair. Some of the people I was sitting with in that room may not make it to their next appointment let alone live to celebrate those milestones with their children. It broke my heart and made me feel very grateful for all of the things I would still be able to enjoy, but I always have a heavy sense of sadness when I see others who have not been as fortunate.

I immediately knew I had no reason to feel sorry for myself and every reason to be thankful. I internalized that and am grateful every day for how fortunate I have been. When someone finds out that I have MS and say, "Oh, I'm so sorry." I always stop them and explain that I don't consider it a negative. Everyone has health problems at some point in their lives. Mine is not terminal and thanks to the protocol, I no longer have to live in fear of what it will do to me next. I live a normal life, and I have dedicated my life to help others do the same. I consider myself extremely blessed, actually. Honestly, what started out as a devastating diagnosis has taught me so many things, starting with never waste a moment!

However, when I was getting that first round of steroids, it would still be years before I found the protocol, and although, I realized that I was very lucky because I would still get to enjoy life, I was fearful of what the next flare would do to me and when it would occur.

After my diagnosis, I had many more hurdles to get over. I still did not fully understand what to expect. I had the intention of heading back to Arizona, but I was afraid that my legs might quit working on the 3,000+ mile trip out there. I did not really understand how unlikely that was, but as you read on these false assumptions just shut down my life for years to come. I was waiting for something to occur at any moment and that paralyzed me.

I had a good job waiting for me with excellent pay and good benefits when I got to Arizona, but I was terrified that if I had blindness or paralysis how would I work? I wanted to start nursing school and decided not to because I feared that the rigors of nursing would not be something my body could not handle, as I expected it to decline. I was told that I would need a physical to get into nursing school and surely when they found out I had MS, I would no longer be a candidate.

In my mind I saw all of the opportunities my disease would preclude me from—or so I thought. I was very open about my diagnosis. I did not want it to be a surprise to people if I suddenly could not walk, etc. I wanted people to remember me as a healthy, vibrant person before the disease began to take away my abilities. I didn't know how or when that would happen but I was afraid of starting nursing school, putting in all that effort only to be surprised with an exacerbation that left me physically unable able to finish school. So I gave up that dream and made some really poor life decisions as a result. This disease was already disabling me mentally. I was closing the door on my life, my dreams and my future.

I began to let fear guide my decision making, and this literally changed the course of my life. It took years for me to realize that my making decisions out of fear did not protect me from heartache and struggles, it only invited more.

For a while, my life revolved around "the shot." I didn't like taking it and I would count the days until I had to go through that process again. The needle was very thin, and when I did it just right it wouldn't hurt, but that wasn't always the case. If I hit a nerve it was painful. If I hit a vessel, I would spew blood across the bathroom. Most injections were okay, but the fear of it made it horrible for me.

The first few weeks I would prepare for hours. I would take ibuprofen beforehand to prevent the side effects that went along with taking the Avonex the first few times. It was suggested that I numb the area about a half hour before I injected. An MS nurse had told me to have pineapple juice to prevent some of the flu-like side effects. I don't know if that worked because I had ibuprofen as well.

I went through this ritual every week. The recommendations were to take the shot before bed, so that I would sleep through the worst of the side effects. I woke up in the middle of the night shaking uncontrollably with the initial shot. I felt like ice. My entire body hurt. I was shaking so badly I could hardly walk to the bathroom and had to do so with a blanket wrapped around me because the air around me felt like it was below zero.

I'm not afraid of needles, but the thought of having to inject myself was a quite a bit scarier than having the nurse do it when I could just look away. It became such a source of stress and dread for me that I got to the point where I just wouldn't do it most weeks. I went for a lot of years rarely taking that shot at all. It was noted that many patients did not take the shot correctly. Due to this, they eventually came out with an auto-injector pen. This pen was a game changer. You didn't see the needle at all. You just pushed the plastic pen onto your leg slightly and pressed the button. The entire thing is over before you know it and usually with little to no pain. I still did not take it every week. I had such a mental block about it. That shot was a reminder of the disease I just wanted to forget, and so I continued for years taking the shot, but very sporadically.

CHAPTER SEVEN

PREGNANCY WITH MS

I was diagnosed in the spring of 2007 and became pregnant with my daughter that fall. The doctors were concerned because I had just turned 36 and they considered anything after 35 a high-risk pregnancy. When I become pregnant there was still a lot of information out there stating that it was not wise to consider pregnancy if you had MS. Well, it was too late for that! So onward! I trusted that if we had any snags they would not be insurmountable.

I did everything in my power to have a healthy pregnancy. I exercised and took very good care of myself. For that reason, my husband nicknamed my daughter the "Whole Foods" baby because I pretty much shopped there for everything for those 9 months. She was super healthy.

It was suggested by the hospital that we have genetic testing to look for anything such as Down's syndrome because of my age. The genetic counselor explained that 80% of the time if a couple learns that they will have a child with Down's syndrome, they choose to terminate the pregnancy. I could not even imagine that for myself. However, I went ahead and had the testing done because if there was a chance we would have a special-needs child, we would have time to make any necessary preparations. My former sister-in-law was developmentally disabled, and we could not imagine the world without her. My only concern was care for the child should my disease progress, so I wanted to have time to make the appropriate arrangements should that be necessary.

However, when our results came back, the odds were astronomically high in favor of a normal outcome. My team of obstetricians were a bit apprehensive about my pregnancy, and neither I nor my neurologist understood why. She assured them that MS would not have any bearing on a pregnancy or delivery. I had a great pregnancy, and my daughter was an extremely healthy baby. There was some fear around anesthesia as I wanted to have an epidural and required a C-section. I was warned that the shocks to my body and pregnancy and birth themselves could cause me to have a relapse. I waited for it to happen, but it never did. She was healthy. I was healthy and after that whole ordeal was over, I brought home a beautiful baby girl, and we went on with life. Incidentally, when she was born, she had one of the biggest, strongest umbilical cords they had ever seen.

I remember they called everyone over to see it. I thought that was funny after all their worry. Today, the thinking surrounding MS and pregnancy is much different. It is thought that pregnancy offers some protection from MS, and that the possibility of relapse increases for a few months after birth, but for most, it is no different than any other pregnancy.

After she was born, I would fear things like losing the use of my arms. What if would I dropped her or somehow hurt her because of my MS? The fact that anything could happen at any time permeated every part of my life. This is how MS disabled me. It injected fear into every area of my life. It stopped me in my tracks mentally. It was like I just went through life frozen in time, gripped with the fear of "what if?"

I went for an MRI once after my daughter was born, and then I stopped going. I decided that the MRIs were not going to tell me anything that I did not already know. I had a new baby, and I was distracted from my MS for once. I was not having any problems, so I just took the position that I was tired of waiting for this disease to do whatever it was going to do. I had given it enough of my life already waiting for whatever may or may not happen. I was going to just live my life.
☐

PREGNANCY ON THE PROTOCOL – GREAT NEWS!

There have been several members come into our group to learn about the protocol so that they can begin once they have their baby. For me, I wish I had been on the protocol when I was pregnant. We are seeing phenomenal results with regard to pregnancy and post-partum in these mothers and babies. Dr. Coimbra recommends 7,000 IU to 10,000 IU of vitamin D daily for pregnant mothers without autoimmune diseases (The importance of Vitamin D during pregnancy). He states that this is absolutely safe during pregnancy, and that it will protect the mother and baby from quite a few problems associated with pregnancy including fertility issues, first-trimester miscarriages and late-pregnancy hypertension and autism.

At the time of the writing of this book, Dr. Coimbra was following about 70 women on vitamin D. They found that these children were born with high psychomotor development. He says, "…literally, gifted children."

In his country, Zika virus has been a problem for quite some time. He states that the placenta of a pregnant woman is able to take in vitamin D and it can block fungi and protozoa from crossing the barrier thus protecting the fetus. So we are finding that there are many reasons to start on vitamin for those who are deficient.

Many times a member will join our group wanting to learn about the protocol so they can start it after their pregnancy. This will not cause you or your baby harm, this is the best time to get on the therapy. You are doing an amazing favor to your child by doing so. Healthy mom and healthy baby!

C H A P T E R   E I G H T

VITAMIN D: THE CONNECTION TO AUTOIMMUNE DISEASE

After every appointment, I would come home and research the latest information on drugs and therapies. I began to notice a trend with vitamin D. I had read about the connection between vitamin D and multiple sclerosis and how the prevalence of multiple sclerosis increased the further you get away from the equator because you weren't getting the vitamin D from the sun that you would get if you were closer to the equator. This made a lot of sense to me.

There were so many studies discussing the role that vitamin D played in the prevention of MS. I surmised that if it could prevent it, maybe it could help it as well. So I had my levels checked. My level was 9. The standard reference range is 20-100 ng/mL, and it is becoming clear that the lower limit should be much higher than 20 ng/mL, as the National Institute of Health, Endocrine Society and Vitamin D Council agree that 40-50 ng/mL is where you no longer have to be concerned about deficiency, unless you are resistant and require even more as is the case in the population with autoimmune diseases (VDCL).

At 9 ng/mL, I was severely deficient. So I begin taking D3 5,000 IU 2 to 3 pills daily several times per week. I did not have a routine. I just made sure I took extra every so often to try to raise my levels. I did not understand the importance of daily dosing at that time. My logic was that since I had no physical disability at this stage, maybe by increasing my levels, I could head it off at the pass. I have taken it ever since.

To this day I think that that's the thing that kept me from having any further disability. I went back to the neurologist in 2011 and there were some new lesions. I got the impression that this was normal progression and to be expected. When I would come back to see my neurologist things would be worse but not a huge concern. She never acted like anything threw up a red flag just that she saw normal progression as was expected. She would ask me whether I had any symptoms, and my answer would always be I have nothing. I feel fine.

☐

A P R I L

In April of 2015, about a year after one of the most stressful events of my life which produced chronic-increasing anxiety, I had went for an MRI. After my MRI, I went to the neurologist for my routine followup and to get the results of my imaging studies. Things had gotten drastically worse. This is the radiology report from that MRI:

```
FINDINGS:
More than 25 enhancing white matter lesions are seen in the
supratentorial compartment, in addition to an enhancing
lesion seen in the left cerebellum and left pons. In
addition, there are about 15 nonenhancing lesions which
were not present in the prior study, for example, in the
left and right frontal regions, image 9-8. In addition, few
of the prior seen lesions appear bigger, for example left
frontal region, image 9-9. The ventricles are normal in
size and position. There is no evidence of significant
brain atrophy. There is no evidence of acute infarct,
intracranial hematoma, extraaxial fluid collection.

There is no cerebellar tonsillar herniation. Expected
arterial flow-voids are present.

The paranasal sinuses, mastoid air cells, and middle ears
are clear. The orbital contents are within normal limits.
No significant osseous or scalp lesions are identified.

IMPRESSION:
1. Multiple new enhancing and nonenhancing lesions,
interval increase in size of few of the lesions which were
present in the prior study.

NOTIFICATION: The significant results of this study were
discussed with, and acknowledged by, Bruen by telephone at
8:40 a.m. on 4/15/2015.
```
☐

It was quite a dramatic decline. So much so that the radiologist felt it necessary to contact neurology to report the results right away. She conveyed to me that she was concerned, but I never realized just how serious it was. She felt like the Avonex was not working anymore. Honestly, I rarely took it at this point, so I just assumed that was the reason. In retrospect, and knowing what I know today about the significant impact that stress has on autoimmune disease, I wholeheartedly believe that it was likely the reason for the rapid acceleration of my disease. I had no idea how serious it was at that point. I had active lesions with nearly every visit so it was disappointing but it did not come as a surprise to me at all.

She said that she would like me to consider Gilenya, Aubagio or Tysabri. I was adamantly opposed to Tysabri. I was aware of the dangers of Tysabri, and I knew that there were deaths associated with progressive multifocal leukoencephalopathy (PML) that had occurred in Tysabri patients. I also knew that it had been taken off the market in 2005 due to the deaths of two patients during the clinical trial and one after the trials had ended.

A year later, Tysabri returned to the market, but with a huge black eye. Many people were afraid of it, and I was one of them. Later, it was discovered that an antibody that a large portion of the population carries to fight off a common virus, the John Cunningham virus (JCV), was partially responsible for the occurrence of PML. The other factor was the administration of immunosuppressant drugs during treatment with Tysabri. The weakening of your immune system gave the opportunistic disease a chance to go in and incur much destruction, sometimes causing worse symptoms than what you may see in MS and was fatal in many instances.

I had a young child at home that needed a healthy mommy, so I just did not feel that the odds were good enough to risk it. In response to this new information regarding the JCV virus, patients would have their JCV titer tested periodically. My issue with Tysabri was that even after they take you off of it, you could continue to have the side effects years later. This just was not acceptable to me. I said I wasn't going to put this toxic drug in my otherwise healthy body.

She once again offered me Gilenya and Aubagio. I declined. I did not feel the other two options were very effective and I did not care for some of the side effects of these drugs either. We went over the pros and cons to each, and honestly I did see benefit to justify taking them other than Tysabri. Tysabri appeared very effective, but at what cost? The cons to Tysabri far outweighed the pros in my mind and I did not feel comfortable with any of the choices.

I explained to her that I rarely took the Avonex, and that I wanted to give that one more chance. I promised her that I would take it faithfully, which I did down to the hour!

Because it takes Avonex about 6 months to reach full efficacy, I would return in the fall for an MRI and then make further decisions at that point. We both agreed that it would be a good idea for me to come back and have an MRI midway through to see where I was at, and so we scheduled and MRI and followup in August. I had lost 20 pounds at this point and had a ways to go. My instructions were to continue my healthy lifestyle and to have 3 days of IV Solu-Medrol infusions to calm down the activity in my brain.

A U G U S T

I returned in August so psyched! I had lost 14 more pounds. I was feeling phenomenal. I had mega energy. I was eating well and exercising. I was pretty sure things would be better. I had been her patient since 2007. I could read her pretty well, and the look on her face when she walked through the door said it all. The radiology report read:

```
FINDINGS:
Numerous supratentorial T2/FLAIR and hyperintense lesions
are noted. Many of these lesions demonstrate peripheral
enhancement. Numerous punctate areas of enhancement
correspond to a smaller FLAIR signal hyperintensities.
Multiple new lesions are noted. The largest new lesion is
seen within the right occipital lobe which demonstrates
faint enhancement along the posterior aspect of the lesion.
Another example of a new lesion is seen within the
posterior aspect of the left temporal lobe (image 8-14).
This demonstrates mild peripheral enhancement. A new lesion
is seen within the left and middle cerebellar peduncle. New
subcortical and lesion with peripheral enhancement is seen
within the right anterior parietal lobe (image 8-6). Mild
global cerebral volume loss is noted. Additionally, several
lesions appear larger in comparison to the prior study.
The ventricles are normal in size and position. No evidence
of extra-axial fluid collection, acute intracranial
hemorrhage, or acute infarct.
Paranasal sinuses, mastoid air cells, and middle ears are
```

clear. No significant calvarial or scalp lesion.

IMPRESSION:
1. Numerous new enhancing supratentorial lesions including a new infratentorial lesion within the left middle cerebellar peduncle compatible with demyelinating disease.
As usual, I was disappointed, but I really had only one choice, and that was to look for the silver lining. I surmised that it was only 3 months in and it took Avonex 6 months to reach full efficacy. I would work even harder and hopefully get better news in November. My instructions were to go for another 3-day round of IV Solu-Medrol, continue my healthy lifestyle and the Avonex.

☐

N O V E M B E R

On November 10th, I had an MRI at 10 a.m. and a neurology appointment at 11:30 a.m. I wanted the results right away so I scheduled them back to back. When I went in to see her on this day, it was obvious that it was difficult for her to break the news to me because I was so hopeful and I had worked so hard to be healthy. She had said to me, "Really Jenn. Cards on the table. You're not having any symptoms?" I wasn't. When she said that, I wondered what she saw on those reports because I got the impression that she thought I may be hiding symptoms. It seemed as though she was surprised that I wasn't having any.

I wonder now that my beginning the 5,000 IU of D a few months back is what had kept me safe and baffled her. Between her questioning and the seriousness she displayed, I knew I could no longer tempt fate, but I still did not want any of those drugs due to their less-than-desirable effects versus efficacy profile. For me, the risk was just too high, and Tysabri was out.

Finally, I had to make a decision, so I chose Aubagio because I felt most comfortable with the safety profile. I could try it and see how things went. Maybe I would do well on it. It seemed like the most logical conservative choice. So I agreed and she said that she would get it started and order a kit for me. I walked out of there defeated. Not only about the drugs, but about my life if I could not stop this thing. I had no more cards up my sleeve. Concerns for my children and our futures were swirling in my head. My brain was not performing at its peak, but in the worry department it was working overtime! What was going to happen to us?

I knew no one could help me but God...so I went to church. I always felt comfort at church and among the people there who wanted to support one another and always could offer encouragement. It was Wednesday night, so that meant prayer meeting. At the end of every meeting they would ask if anyone needed to come up for prayer. I never went up for stuff like that, but this night I knew only God could help. I went up there and told them what was going on. Everyone gathered around me and placed their hands on me and began to pray. I am a Christian, and I believe that God can heal. I don't believe the answer is always yes though.

For myself, I felt like, "Why would God heal me? I'm not really doing anything special where I am of use to him." This was a warped perspective, but at the time, it was how I believed...sort of like I had not done anything to earn it. After I got better and began the group, I relayed this story with one of the group members, Brandon, who I befriended and told him how I didn't know why God would choose to heal me because I was not doing anything to help people. He said to me, "But maybe he knew you would." He asked how it felt to stumble into my destiny. That changed my whole perspective. I had never thought of it that way.

In my mind, I could not fathom anyone not wanting to grab every suffering patient out there and drag them to the nearest protocol doctor. I was compelled to tell anyone who would listen. Think of the lives we could change! Not only patients, but their families who love them. Maybe small children who depend on them. It could bring blessings to so many people. I was on fire and I could not stop!

After I was diagnosed, I spent a lot of time learning about the disease, and honestly looking for a miracle, but once the initial shock wore off and I felt like I had educated myself about MS, I rarely followed the new drugs and treatments that came out. I would get excited by headlines that read, "Possible Cure for MS" only to find by the end of the article that a cure was "still years away."

The only time I would do any research would be immediately after my neurology visits when I was once again reminded that there was nothing that could be done. In one of these sessions I came across an article that discussed a very strong correlation between MS and vitamin D. I was intrigued, and so on this evening, after church, I decided to see if any new advances or discoveries had been made in this area. I always Googled for information, but I had recently learned how informative YouTube could be and I much preferred watching videos to reading.

I begin to look up vitamin D and found videos of patients discussing a doctor that had treated them with very high doses of vitamin D. Because this doctor was Brazilian, most of these patients spoke Portuguese and I was unable to understand the videos. However there were about four or five videos that had English subtitles. The first video showed a young man in his 20s who explained that he, over the course of several years, became very ill with the inability to control many functions, and had difficulty with walking and weakness among other things. He was so ill he could not travel to visit one of the few protocol doctors available at the time, so the protocol doctor sent him a prescription.

The young man got markedly better with a resolution of symptoms. Today he will speak to whomever is interested in learning more about the protocol and find out how they too can halt their disease the way he did. I found a video of Dr. Coimbra and sat for an hour and a half and listening to everything he said on the edge of my seat in tears because I realized that there were too many patients telling the same story for this to be anything other than the real deal. They weren't selling anything. These weren't well choreographed videos. These were just regular people telling their stories.

My first question was the question most people ask: "If this is such a great treatment how come the world doesn't know about it?" Once I got the answer to that question and felt comfortable that this was a legitimate therapy, I started talking to anybody who might be knowledgeable about vitamin D and pulled up every bit of information I possibly could. I was shocked to find that there were years and years' worth of studies showing that vitamin D does indeed affect MS in amazing ways.

The most concentrated groups of these patients could be found on Facebook. I joined every Facebook group I could, but most of them were international groups because the therapy had started in Brazil and rippled out from there. These groups were extremely helpful. They had lots of English-speaking members who were more than happy to share what they had learned with me. I had gotten in touch with this young man who had such a remarkable recovery. I wanted to talk to him because I was terrified at the notion of stopping my medication in favor of a natural treatment. After all, I really did not have much faith in healing through diet and supplements and a part of me still doubted that they were going to be that helpful, but I was about to find out that the joke was on me! It sounded so strange and irresponsible but I was looking at proof. I was seeing patients over and over and over saying this halted their MS, and in some cases this reversed their symptoms.

Because I was still symptom free, and had no idea just how bad my MRIs were at the time, I felt like it was a risk that I was willing to take. I'm not sure that if I had realized the actual severity of my progression if I would have felt comfortable enough to make the same decision. I'm thankful I did not know because my story may have come out drastically different. I posted this in one of the groups:

Good morning everyone, I'm struggling with a dilemma. My Avonex is not working. I have had a new enhancing lesion on the last 3 MRIs. I've had MS since 2007 with no disabilities, thankfully. I don't care for my choices due to PML risks (call it paranoia, but I'm just being honest). I agreed to Aubagio if she would agree to run the labs for the vitamin D protocol. However after reading up on Aubagio, I really just don't want to dump anymore junk in my otherwise healthy body. I have been on D3 but only 20,000 IU. I think I'm going to try this because I really feel good about it (vitamin D protocol). I would like to hear from people who have been on it and have (and have not had) success so I can make a solid decision. This is so hard. I would really appreciate it because right now, I'm a little scared. Thanks.

This young man told me not to be afraid and that it really was okay, and went on to explain everything that he could about the protocol to me. I told him that I didn't think I could afford a trip to Brazil, and he said, "There is the new doctor in the states." He gave me the number to an ophthalmology clinic. That sounded highly suspect to me, but I believe in giving everyone an opportunity, so I called the clinic and spoke to a very nice gentleman and asked him "How does an ophthalmologist wind up treating neurological disorders?" He sort of laughed and explained that his wife is from Brazil and she was familiar with the protocol, and that he had a family member with MS. He said they started the family member on the protocol and today the family member is fine.

Hearing that from a doctor was a great comfort to me and that settled it. I made an appointment with this doctor and flew to visit him. I was a little nervous about what I was going to walk into. Part of me was concerned that I was going to wind up in front of a rundown doctor's office on the bad side of town. However it could not have been any further from my expectations. It was a lovely area. The office was pristine and beautiful. The staff was extremely professional and accommodating.

The doctor was meticulous and professional. I was impressed. My appointment lasted about 2- 1/2 to 3 hours. I had to bring a set of baseline labs and I have never had a more thorough medical history taken in my life then I had that day. We talked a lot about my health, my family history and my stress level which is very closely related to autoimmune diseases. I was given a thorough neurological exam exactly like the one that my neurologist gives me for my yearly routine follow-up. It was apparent I was in very good hands. When I walked out of the office that day I felt so confident in this therapy, all I could do with count down the days until that MRI. I was told not to expect too much on MRI for probably seven months to a year. Because I didn't have any physical disability to speak of, I didn't expect to notice much change and realized that I had to be patient for quite some time before I would know if this would actually work or not.

☐

NURSING SCHOOL

In 2014, when I had that major event in my life that caused me so much stress, I signed up for college courses in an attempt to distract myself from it. I decided college would keep my mind so busy, I would not have time to even think about this other thing. So in the months prior to that first discouraging MRI, I had signed up for college courses.

I wanted to go to nursing school. I had come to the realization that I had wasted too much time and I needed to work double duty to make up for all of that time I had lost. I signed up for the prerequisites for nursing with the ultimate goal of becoming a nurse practitioner and working with veterans. I had worked with brain-injured veterans years ago and I really loved that job. I wanted to give back, and if my MS got worse…well it's hard to focus on your problems when you're working daily with a population who have seen the worst that life can throw at you and still manage to move forward with a good attitude. I admired them so much for their courage and perseverance under unimaginable circumstances.

When I was in high school, I really did not do well. Family problems stole my motivation and I was apathetic. I was a bit intimidated by college due to my less-than-stellar performance in high school. I always tested very high, but my grades did not reflect that, so I was concerned that I would not make the grade—literally and figuratively—in college. I was surprised to find the coursework surprisingly easy.

I was running a household, a business, homeschooling my daughter and attending college full time—successfully! Many people said I needed to slow down, but I enjoyed the fast pace. I was in love with academia. I easily maintained a 4.0 through the first several semesters and then something happened. I was studying as hard—if not harder—than I ever had, but remembering less. I spent hours and hours going over my work and I noticed in math, I was unable to remember the series of steps to take to work the equations. I loved anatomy. I found everything about it fascinating. I had heard horror stories about anatomy, but I think the fact that I enjoyed it so much and was blessed with an awesome professor made it easy to like. A friend of my said, switch to this professor he's great. Even the university students came over to the junior college to get in his class if they could not get into his class at the university. He taught at both places.

Somehow I got in. It took me all of 5 minutes to realize what all the fuss was about. He was humorous but demanded excellence. I loved it! He had a way of leading you to the answer in a way that forced you to think about it without feeling pressured. You enjoyed it. He was engaging and just one of the students. He discussed with you and did not talk at you.

Being a homeschool mom, I tried to learn his teaching style to apply to my homeschool. So all of this made the class a pleasure to attend. However, as time went on, I noticed that no matter how much I studied I could not retain it. I was so frustrated with myself. I tried to hide the fact that I was struggling by joking around, but honestly I was really concerned.

The vision in my left eye began to get blurry and I had to go get glasses because we would look at a lot of things that were very tiny and I just could not make them out. Everything was collapsing. I put so much time and effort into these classes and I was bombing! I knew the blurry vision was probably MS related because I had eye pain in my left eye before and that is the eye that was giving me problems again.

The memory issues I just chalked up to running so hard that year, except physically I felt the best I had ever felt. I was eating very well, exercising, and getting plenty of rest. There were some extenuating circumstances that were causing me quite a bit as stress however. That's the only thing I could think of. I never even thought it was MS related. I ended up in tears on more than one occasion because I was giving my all, and I just could not remember all of those hours of studying.

When we were studying the skeletal system, we began to discuss vitamin D, so I brought my professor some information about the protocol and asked him what he thought. He said, "You could die." I asked him why and he brought up vitamin D toxicity. We discussed it for a bit and he said if I had anything else that I would like him to read over, that he would be willing to do so. I brought him one more paper, but I was doing so poorly in his class by this point, that I didn't think he thought I took it seriously and so I was a bit intimidated to talk to him anymore which was a shame because I really wanted to pick his brain endlessly!

One particular afternoon, I had an hour between lecture and lab where we had just discussed oligodendrocytes, the cells in the brain responsible for creating the myelin sheath around the neurons of the brain. We had just been taught that the problem with MS was that even though oligodendrocytes created myelin, they were not very effective at it, and they did not produce enough to regenerate myelin well enough to repair damage incurred by multiple sclerosis. I was sitting in the car scrolling through vitamin D articles when came across a brand new study by the University of Cambridge that stated:

"Researchers, from the MS Society Cambridge Centre for Myelin Repair, identified that the 'vitamin D receptor' protein pairs with an existing protein, called the RXR gamma receptor, already known to be involved in the repair of myelin, the protective sheath surrounding nerve fibres.
By adding vitamin D to brain stem cells where the proteins were present, they found the production rate of oligodendrocytes (myelin making cells) increased by 80%. When they blocked the vitamin D receptor to stop it from working, the RXR gamma protein alone was unable to stimulate the production of oligodendrocytes." (Cambridge)

By this time, I had already booked my flight to visit the doctor who would start me on the protocol. I could have jumped out of my car and danced around the parking lot! I was on the right track. Everything in me knew that I was on the right track pursuing this protocol. I tell the group that this is my favorite study—this is the reason. It just confirmed everything I suspected.

Vitamin D IS THE KEY!!!!

C H A P T E R   N I N E

"OH MY GOSH! IT'S WORKING!"

Several weeks later I would become the first patient in the US to visit the first protocol doctor in the US. It was pretty exciting! Once the labs came back, I began the protocol.

One afternoon a month or so after beginning the protocol, I was cleaning in my office and came across my glasses. It was funny because I had completely forgotten needed my glasses. I had dropped anatomy because I was struggling so badly. Anatomy was the only place I used them so I had not thought about them in weeks. It occurred to me that I had forgotten about them. The same glasses that a few months before would cause panic if I left for class without them!

And that's when it hit me. I have not thought about them because I'm not having any blurry vision anymore! I had this cramp in my foot that I could reproduce if I pointed my toes that I was pretty sure was an MS symptom. So I immediately pointed my toes and I could not make it cramp up. At that moment, I yelled, "Oh, my gosh! It's working!"

I immediately called my doctor and asked her if we could get an MRI. She said yes, and on June 7, 2016 I had my first MRI after beginning the protocol. Later than morning, I went to see my doctor. I sat in her office so nervous. I had a little discussion with myself that went something like:

Now Jenn, you know that the doctors told you that you shouldn't expect to see anything on MRI before about 7 to 12 months. If there's anything bad on the MRI, you need to remind yourself that you've only been doing this for a couple of months and it's not uncommon to see some residual progression until the vitamin D has been optimized. You made a commitment to one year so if the news is bad you're not going to cry, you're going to stand up tall and walk out of here, knowing that this is going to help and you've got a ways to go yet.

I could usually read her when she came in, but on this day I could not read her. She said that it had been a busy day for her and so we would just look at my images together. When she opened the images, where there were white spots before…there was nothing! Like someone had just erased them! They were completely blank. We both just sat there with our jaws on the floor. She remarked several times "that's impressive." I'm not sure who was more stunned. But I do know that we high-fived, and I did end up crying, but not out of disappointment…FOR ONCE, I walked out of there so happy! I never had an MRI that did not have active lesions. My previous MRIs said I had numerous new lesions. And for the first time in 10 years there was no disease activity. My lesions were still there, but all of them inactive!

My radiology report read:

```
IMPRESSION:
Multiple bilateral supratentorial T2/FLAIR hyperintense
lesions compatible with known multiple sclerosis, with no
evidence of active disease on today's exam. Probable
interval new non-enhancing lesion in the right parasagittal
frontal lobe (image 8-6, 9-6).
```

It was early on in my treatment and I was on an extremely conservative test dose, but I had no activity. I had a "probable" new lesion, but all other lesions were inactive. Considering my previous reports, this was truly amazing!

My doctor asked if I was still taking the medication. And I told her that I never took it because I was concerned that if my MRI came back good it could be said that it was the medication at work and not the vitamin D. At that, she said once again "That's impressive!" For the first time ever I left her office and did not have to go get a Solu-Medrol infusion. My instructions this time we're to just keep doing what I was doing.

I could have skipped out of that office I was so happy! I was laughing. I was crying. I was telling everybody that knew what I was doing. I told my family. I told my friends. I told the ladies in the lab! It was one of the best days of my life. It was the beginning of my new life, and slowly the gears of hope began to turn again…that steel door that I never thought could be open swung open and I was running through it as fast as I could! I had my life back. No more MS. No more bad MRIs. A future!!!!

Once I came back down to earth I started thinking, "I have to let people know about this!" I told the group that had been helping me, and I told the young man who encouraged me to try it. I realized we didn't have a group for English speaking people. So I took what little bit of knowledge I had about Facebook and started a Facebook group, not having any expectations of what was to come. Before I knew it, we had a steady stream of people.

That was June of 2016. That was 16 months ago, today we have 5000+ members from every country in the world and our numbers are growing exponentially. I could've never anticipated our success. I have met some of the most remarkable people in the last year and a half since our group began. We have seen countless people turn their lives around. We have seen skeptical people hesitantly try the protocol and come back just beside themselves upon experiencing the same success I experienced. We have brought new doctors on board.

We have worked really hard to provide every tool possible to help members have success on the protocol. There are a small percentage of members who for some reason or another don't realize the full benefit of the protocol, but we constantly work with them as much as we possibly can to try and sort this out with them. We never give up on members. We will not leg you go.

The group has become a giant family of supportive people who are traveling down this road together. We have people posting videos of their progress and it's just amazing to watch and cheer them on. My Messenger, text, email, and telephone are rarely quiet; ringing, buzzing, dinging and beeping throughout the day with patients asking questions or new patients wanting to learn how they can begin. I absolutely love what I do.

The gratitude I feel for the privilege to be a part of this just can't fully be expressed in words. As our group has grown this has become my life's calling. I said originally that if this works I will shout it from the rooftops to anyone who will listen. I was very afraid of having my face and information out there on the Internet but today I'm proud to be able to share this with people, and that fear that has long been put to rest. We are constantly looking for new innovative ways to reach out and share this amazing therapy with as many people as we possibly can.

CHAPTER TEN

THE GROUP

The Facebook Group, Coimbra Vitamin D Protocol for MS & Autoimmune Diseases is a beautiful illustration serendipity. There is something very special, I would say divine, about our coming together.

I cannot tell you how many people have said to me. I feel there is a connection here that brought us all together, or we are all on the same wavelength. We have been told many times that we are the nicest group that members have been in. I believe that is because we have a mutual understanding of the significance of our fortune and the gravity of our responsibility to those that will come after us.

Our group works very hard to remain credible in an environment where many may view us as just another fringe health group. What sets us apart, however, is proof. Thousands of patients who are well. Doctors who are seeing this for themselves and beginning to join us.

Our numbers are growing, and as the world witnesses others getting well on this protocol, it is beginning to sit up and pay attention. I hope that this book is another step in that direction. I heard it said one time that just because you don't believe in gravity, it is not going to change the result if you jump out a window.

To those who are ill and unsure, we can provide you with testimony after testimony of the amazing power of this treatment. My sincere wish is that you will come talk to us and get started. The sooner you seek treatment the better your outcome. Please don't wait.

TESTIMONY OF BOO BARKSDALE

My name is Boo Barksdale and I will have been on the Coimbra vitamin D3 protocol to treat MS for 9 months on November 30th, 2017. I'm 60 years old with primary progressive multiple sclerosis (PPMS). I discovered the protocol while reading a comment on a blog on an MS website in December of 2016 after following a link to protocol information. I located quite a bit of protocol information online, and I began researching vitamin D as much as I could. I Also found Ana Claudia Domene's book, 'Multiple Sclerosis and (lots of) Vitamin D', which has lots of good information, and it has many links to more information and videos in the back of the book. I highly recommend it.

I had taken 2000 IU of vitamin D daily for a couple of years before my MS diagnosis. As I read more books on vitamin D and I increased the amount I was taking from 2000 IU to 5000 IU daily and then to 15,000 IU. I was desperate to feel better and see a reduction of symptoms, and I felt like I had found the path to healing and hope with the Coimbra protocol.

With the holistic practices I participated in when I found the protocol, I felt like I was treading water, but needed something more. At 15,000 IU of vitamin D, I began to see some noticeable improvements in my energy level and mobility. I also saw reduced spasticity. My legs and arms felt less heavy.
I was still ambulatory, but I could see a slow, steady decline and progression of symptoms. I was 59 years old and I knew time was not on my side. These small improvements encouraged me and gave me the confidence to discuss the protocol with my primary care doctor because I needed assistance in getting the necessary labs done in order to begin the protocol. I was also taking a B complex supplement and vitamin B 12; at the time guided with the help of a local nutritionist that works with elite athletes and has a nutrition business.

After a previous primary care doctor that I had seen for many years told me repeatedly that he thought my symptoms were all related to my thyroid, he began to sound like a broken record and so I sought another opinion. I do also have Hashimoto's which was well controlled with thyroid medication prior to my MS diagnosis.

The second doctor being much more methodical and considered in his approach, ordered an MRI which led to my diagnosis. It took me about 6 years of living with MS symptoms continuously before finally being diagnosed. My earliest recognizably-undeniable symptom goes back to 2004 with slurred speech. A CT scan at that time came back inconclusive and I ignored other minor symptoms like minor tingling and occasional numbness, or my foot not working properly after I'd had an alcoholic beverage.

I was diagnosed with MS in October 2014 at age 57. My future, as described by the medical community, was very limited, but that was their description, not mine. I had other plans. After diagnosis, I did everything I could to eliminate stress and improve my diet and simplify my lifestyle. I followed my intuition. There are many sources of nutritional information for MS patients so I won't address nutrition here.

I obtained the labs and had my first consultation for the protocol in late February of 2017. I began the protocol on March 1, 2017. I was still walking, but using a walking stick some of the time, and feeling my right side becoming significantly weaker than my left. My biggest fear was losing mobility because I have a 13-year-old daughter whom I want to walk down the aisle. Because of my age and the slow steady progression of symptoms over a period of many years without interruption, my diagnosis was soon modified to primary progressive, PPMS by my neurologist. At the time of my diagnosis there were no FDA-approved treatment options for PPMS. My only option in the traditional medical community at the time of diagnosis, was treatment with IV steroids, which did slow down the symptoms for a period of a few months, but they returned unabated. My primary symptoms at the time of diagnosis were debilitating fatigue, balance issues, muscle weakness, and my mobility was beginning to become seriously impaired. Coordination, and clear thinking were also problematic. I could only be active, standing, bending, kneeling and walking any distance for a short time, maybe 15 minutes. But I did participate in an exercise research program through the University of Texas for 6 months with a personal trainer getting her PhD in nursing, studying the cognitive effects of exercise on MS patients, and I learned the value of exercise in helping deal with MS. The one thing I had going for me was that I was a distance runner for 40 years. I didn't run my first marathon until I was forty one, and looking back I may have had MS then and not known it. That was in 1998.

While my employer at the time of my diagnoses was stellar, and worked with me to make adjustments to my job position. I had to stop working because stress from job-related issues and warm or hot weather (I worked mostly outdoors in central Texas) aggravated my symptoms, and I stopped working in June 2015 right before my 58th birthday. Stress from my job was the main aggravator of symptoms that I could identify at the time, and as Dr. Coimbra advises, eliminating stress is a key component to success on the protocol. I have chosen to treat my MS holistically because there were and are no other viable treatment options for PPMS and the holistic approach aligned with my philosophy for living and addressing illness. Other important elements of my practice for returning to health in addition to the protocol include nutrition, exercise, (yoga and walking), acupuncture, chiropractic, massage, energy therapy and any other approach that I've been able to research and found valuable. I also practice meditation and creative visualization, and I use a CBD oil to maintain a sense of calm and mental balance as well as prevent anxiety. There's no THC in the product I use (7 CBD). There's a lot of science behind the CBD. Each one of these approaches provide benefits, but I had not found the lynch pin to my approach to treating MS until I discovered Dr. Coimbra's vitamin D3 protocol. I would like to point out that the return to health on any path is not a straight line. Ups and downs should be expected. Being prepared for variables makes incorporating adjustments along the way easier. For the first 12 weeks on the Coimbra protocol things went smoothly and I saw slow, steady improvements, then I felt like I plateaued. My initial dose of vitamin D was 50,000 IU daily. I took it in the standard form of vitamin D in one capsule. I also took a compounded MS supplement with some of the other recommended vitamins and minerals selenium, chromium etc., and the magnesium in addition to the vitamin D. I have learned since starting the protocol that there are significant differences between types of B2 vitamins (regular and pre-activated), and there are many different types of magnesium that address different areas of the body in different ways. There are also significant differences between different brands of vitamins, and how individuals respond to them. Some product brands work better than others too. At the end of June, I could walk up to a mile occasionally, but usually it was a half mile, and I was very encouraged.

Then in mid-July I had a significant setback. I saw the biggest setback in my walking. My muscles did not respond well and muscle fatigue increased also. I had lower energy too, although it was still much better than before, I started the protocol, so I felt sure the protocol was working, but I knew something was out of adjustment. I was confident I was on the right track, but I needed assistance making adjustments to the supplements I was taking. I didn't know where to turn as the protocol doctor I initially consulted with became extremely busy because of the increased popularity of the protocol and we were unable to communicate. Through the North American Facebook protocol page a prayer was answered. I had prayed for guidance. And an answer came in a phone call that started in a conversation on a Sunday afternoon. A Facebook friend, John Otwell contacted me about a question unrelated to my setback. John wanted to speak to me about a comment I had made a few months earlier in a post about the mind healing before the body. We spoke on the telephone, he in Missouri and I in Texas. I related my experience that prompted my comment. John asked how I was doing, and I told him about the setback I had encountered. John encouraged me as he always does with his positive attitude and steady personality, delivered with humor. We encouraged each other and I hung up, I thought that was the end of it.

The next morning at 9 o'clock my phone rang and it was John again, he said he had spoken to his protocol advisor about me and that is advisor wanted to speak with me, and thought he might know what was happening with me. I was stunned that all of this was happening for my benefit without any involvement from me. I emailed the advisor and received a phone call the next day. He reviewed the supplements I was taking and suggested changes. After I received the new supplements I saw improvements in a few days. The improvements were limited because I had miss understood I needed to be taking three different types of magnesium. I was only taking one type of magnesium. After another adjustment I saw more improvement.

At this time I was still only taking 50,000 IU of vitamin D and all of the standard type. I had tried micellized D but didn't notice enough improvement to switch to the micellized D, and it is a more expensive product.

In late July 2017 I had a new set of labs done. Inadvertently I had consumed some dairy by eating ricotta cheese in vegetarian lasagna more than once. My total calcium came back slightly above range. I needed to have my calcium and PTH retested.
My PTH was suspiciously low at 5. It turned out the B complex vitamin I was taking contained biotin and it caused a false number on the PTH lab.

It took a several weeks to get retested as I was on vacation traveling with my wife. When the new labs came back my PTH was 21 and the calcium was in range at 10.1. I'm now taking 62,000 IU of D; part of it micellized, part regular. I'm feeling better than any time in over 2 years and I'm continuing to gain traction with my improvements.

My energy level is normal, I don't stop during the day to rest unless I want to.

I'm noticing better strength in my muscles during yoga, and my walking is also slowly improving too. I can walk more than a half mile no problem, and I'm pushing for more constantly.

What all of this illustrates to me is the combined strength of our common goal brought together through social media on Facebook to help each of us help each other, and the power of community with a common goal. I didn't get where I am alone.

We are a grassroots effort to overcome MS through the power of social media. Through the Facebook group we are providing information to the medical community so more medical practitioners can be educated about the benefits available through vitamin D and Dr. Coimbra's protocol for MS and autoimmune issues, and doctors are seeking out information through the Facebook group. I'm glad to be able to provide my personal information and story to add one more voice to the chorus spreading the word about the Coimbra protocol.

There is no doubt that this works and every day provides more evidence. My most significant improvement in addition to walking is regaining the ability to tap my right foot. It may seem like a small thing, but I noticed that ability disappear in July and now it's back. I could do it when I saw the neurologist the beginning of June and then the ability to tap my right foot left during my set back in July which may have started after starting pre-activated B2 which I was cautioned about, meaning my vitamin D level was high at 257 ng/dl, so there was a lot of vitamin D3 sitting unused in my blood.

The pre-activated b2 caused stress to my system as it's more powerful than the standard b2. When my body tried to convert and use too much vitamin d3, it didn't like it.

I had to back off the pre-activated b2 a bit and give myself time to adjust.

In early November as I adjusted, I noticed I had regained the ability to tap my right foot, another success. With the success and confidence I've gained on Dr. Coimbra's vitamin D protocol, I'm now applying to participate in Spring 2018 Oceans of Hope sailing cruise for patients with MS in Croatia, cruising islands in The Adriatic Sea. None of this would be possible without the protocol.

Today I consider myself the person doing the thing they said couldn't be done, smiling in the face of a big challenge. We are all that person. Thank you to everyone that supports and works on the protocol.

ABOUT THE AUTHOR

JENNIFER BUTLER is the founder of the Coimbra Vitamin D Protocol for MS & Autoimmune Diseases Facebook group. She lives with her family in the foothills of the Blue Ridge Mountains of central Virginia. She loves to educate doctors and patients about the amazing effects of vitamin D in hopes of one day eradicating autoimmune diseases forever.

Learn more about Jennifer at: www.CoimbraVitaminDProtocol.com

WORKS CITED

n.d. 23 Oct. 2017.
⟨http://www.vivo.colostate.edu/hbooks/pathphys/endocrine/othere
ndo/vitamind.html⟩.

Oct. 2000. Web. 4 Nov. 2017.
⟨https://www.researchgate.net/publication/12339485_Autoimmune
_diseases_A_leading_cause_of_death_among_young_and_middle-
aged_women_in_the_United_States⟩.

n.d. Web. 4 Nov 2017. ⟨https://www.healthline.com/health/multiple-
sclerosis/facts-statistics-infographic⟩.

Biophysics, Archives of Biochemistry and. "Where is the Vitamin D
Receptor?" *Archives of Biochemistry and Biophysics* 523.1 (2012): 123-133.
Web. 5 Nov. 2017.

Calvo, Dr Francisco. *Interview with Dr Cicero Galli Coimbra.* 7 Mar. 2016. Web.
27 Sept. 2017. ⟨https://www.youtube.com/watch?v=-
IYfBNOe7p8&t=1702s⟩.

Cicero Galli Coimbra, MD, PhD. *Coimbra, vitamina D e patologie autoimmuni*
Leonardo Rubini. 17 Apr. 2014. 28 Aug 2017.
⟨https://www.youtube.com/watch?v=hOfO29rL-gI&t=675s⟩.

The importance of Vitamin D during pregnancy. 27 Aug. 2017. 20 10 2017.
⟨https://www.youtube.com/watch?v=Ivz_DzW4z5U⟩.

The Lancet Neurology. "Health-care use before a first demyelinating event
suggestive of a multiple sclerosis prodrome: a matched cohort
study." *The Lancet Neurology* 16.2 (2017): 445-451. Web.
⟨http://www.thelancet.com/journals/laneur/article/PIIS1474-
4422(17)30076-5/fulltext⟩.

Made in the USA
Lexington, KY
21 January 2018